I0441088

Lecture Reprint Number 6

How To Build A Better Body From Your Kitchen

by Bernard Jensen, D.C., N.D.,
Nutritionist

Revised and edited by Jon D. Jensen

ACKNOWLEDGEMENTS

I acknowledge and give thanks to Betty Norlin for being such a wonderful friend and for continually encouraging me and assisting me on my book writing/editing journey. Author of *"Our Bodies: The Optimal Design."* www.bettynorlin.com www.whatisholistichealth.com

I acknowledge and give thanks to Daylin Anderson, B.S. in Psychology, Cognitive and Behavioral Neuroscience/Human Development, for editing and compiling information for this lecture reprint booklet series. Daylin is a cherished friend who typed up many of these booklets for me and made it possible to finish this project. She truly is my inspiration and muse.

I acknowledge and give thanks to Gary and Jeanne Nichols. They have given to me their expertise in editing and marketing as well as assisting me with my grandfather's videos taking them from video to DVD. They have always supported me whether it was creating an office space, writing, or giving lectures. Thank you both!

COPYRIGHT

Copyright @ 2019 by Jon D. Jensen

All rights reserved. No part of this book may be reproduced, stored, or transmitted by any means – whether auditory, graphic, mechanical, or electronic – without written permission of both publisher and author, except in the case of brief excerpts used in critical articles and reviews. Unauthorized reproduction of any part of this work is illegal and punishable by law.

Because of the dynamic nature of the Internet, any web addresses or links contained in this book may have changed since publication and may no longer be valid.

Paperback ISBN: 9781089887591

DISCLAIMER

Any information given in this book is not intended to be taken as a replacement for medical advice. Any person with a condition requiring medical attention should consult a qualified health professional.

INTRODUCTION

My name is Jon Jensen and I have been involved in the holistic health field for many years. I have published a nutrition book, "A Simple Guide to Healthy Living" as a way to communicate with people outside my client base with information I feel is key to a healthy life. It is available on Amazon or through my website, www.jensenholistichealth.com

I've wanted to publish these health booklets for many years. My intention for editing, revising, and publishing my grandfather's 21 lecture reprint booklets is rooted in my desire to continue his legacy of teaching right living through health and nutrition. Dr. Bernard Jensen spent his lifetime helping others to achieve health through education and his writing, and I feel strongly that the message is needed now more than ever.

I always marveled that my grandfather, Dr. Bernard Jensen, could write so many books and still travel, receive numerous awards, teach classes on Iridology, rejuvenation/regeneration, and tissue cleansing. These lecture reprints are the product of his first lectures, typed up and stapled into booklets and originally sold for ninety-nine cents each. Thus, the beginning of a pattern where he would write and self-publish many books over his lifetime. He did end up publishing books with a couple different publishing companies, but most of his work was self-published.

DR. BERNARD JENSEN, PH.D., N.D., D.C.

One of the greatest healers the world has ever known. Dr. Bernard Jensen spent over 60 years as a pioneer in the holistic health field, helping to pave the way for the alternative health revolution that we are now experiencing.

Dr. Jensen began his career at the West Coast Chiropractic College where Bernard became the youngest chiropractor in the state of California. He traveled extensively in search of health knowledge, a search that led him to over 65 countries to observe the lifestyles of the people and their various ways of eating. Each place provided a different health secret.

Throughout his career, Dr. Jensen wrote and published over 60 books. After working with over 350,000 patients, Dr. Jensen firmly believed that nutrition is the greatest single therapy to be applied in the holistic healing arts and that "We must treat the patient, not just the disease."

Born on March 25, 1908, to parents of Danish descent, Eugen and Anna Jensen, Jorgen Bernard Jensen was raised in Stockton, California, then a small rural town in one of the richest agricultural valleys of the state. The unexpected death of his mother at age 29 from tuberculosis and consumption left three children to be raised by their father, Eugen Jensen, who was a chiropractor. Very little has been written about Bernard's early life growing up in Stockton, his brother and sister, and a few comments in lectures he made about his father who was mentioned as very strict and analytical.

Early in life, young Bernard displayed the qualities needed for his future work. His penchant for being an analytical, critical, serious perfectionist blended with his sensitive, competitive, spiritual-minded personality to arm him with an unusual perspective that opened the doors to the unconventional life he was soon to enter. But before that path was firmly set, several intense learning experiences occurred which determined the direction he was to take.

Being his own worst obstacle, restless and never satisfied, he would rather study and read a book than eat or sleep. His father was a chiropractor, and young Bernard followed in his path. When he was 18 years old, Bernard entered the West Coast Chiropractic College in Oakland, California. During his four years of study, Bernard burned the midnight oil while holding down as many as two outside jobs simultaneously. The strain was immense. The capacity to push forward and the ability to persevere doggedly toward a goal were firmly established, but there was a price to pay. Bernard supported himself by working at a dairy in his spare time, and the long hours of work and study, along with poor food habits, took a heavy toll on Bernard's health. After receiving his diploma in 1929, Dr. Bernard Jensen went into practice, opening his first office in Oakland, California. He focused intently on the task of his calling which was to offer a helping hand to those suffering and in need. Dr. Bernard Jensen's devotion was complete, the hours long, his personal needs forgotten. By this time, the sacrificing of many years began to demand attention. His health began to fail. A Medical Doctor diagnosed his condition as bronchiectasis, an often-fatal lung condition, with no known cure at the time. "There is nothing I can do for you," he was told.

The young man refused to give up, searching out a Seventh Day Adventist Medical Doctor who taught him basic nutritional principles, told Dr. Bernard Jensen to leave junk food alone and promptly presented him with a maintenance program involving natural health that emphasized the return to a pure, natural, and whole foods regimen. Following this program brought excellent results. Dr. Bernard Jensen was soon on the way back to health and renewed vitality. A great turning point had occurred. To be able to study nutrition and discover the laws of right living became his burning desire. Dr. Bernard Jensen turned the experience of what he learned from the Seventh Day Adventist Medical Doctor about the holistic approach into helping his patients get better and teaching them how to prevent themselves from getting sick. Dr. Bernard Jensen began taking breathing exercises with Thomas Gaines, once an instructor for the New York City Police Department. Slowly, and over a period of time, his health returned, and his lungs eventually healed completely.

Using this knowledge in working with his patients the results were dramatic and effective. Dr. Bernard Jensen's attention was now riveted in this direction. Natural therapeutics became his healing mode, setting the pattern for the rest of his life. He began to travel in search of more knowledge and information.

After Dr. Bernard Jensen opened his first office in Oakland, California, in 1929, he later moved to Los Angeles and expanded his practice to include branch offices at Long Beach and Santa Monica, with several chiropractors working under him. Such success had not come about overnight. In Chicago, Dr. Bernard Jensen took his post-graduate work at the National Chiropractic College and later from the Los Angeles Chiropractic College closer to home. Upon returning to California, he began an intensive study and investigation of something he was recently just learning about, the subject of iridology.

Dr. Bernard Jensen used Rocine's work as the basis for the programs used in his sanitariums—first a 25-bed sanitarium in San Leandro, California, then others in Ben Lomand and Alta Dena, and finally an 85-bed sanitarium at Hidden Valley Health Ranch in Escondido, California. The sanitariums were quite successful, demonstrating the effectiveness of Rocine's ideas in working with patients. It was the Hidden Valley Health Ranch in Escondido that provided the greatest opportunity for applying the rules of right living. People in search of health and rejuvenation came to the ranch from all over the world to learn the principles that Dr. Bernard Jensen believed in, practiced, and taught.

Proper nutrition, together with sunshine, rest, exercise, fresh air, and positive attitudes helped thousands of patients at Dr. Bernard Jensen's sanitariums leave behind the symptoms of chronic diseases that they had developed.

Patients came from all over the world, came to stay at his sanitariums, others for outpatient consultations, and still others to attend his classes in rejuvenation and food studies. Thousands of New Zealanders formed clubs to follow his dietetic advice, filling out the over 350,000 people he reached, accumulated over the years. He acquired a multitude of experiences from these people individually and in group studies, acquiring information and summing it up for use in his healing work and writing.

Dr. Bernard Jensen visited the Hunza Valley, where disease, doctors, dentists, and hospitals were practically nonexistent and where there were no jails, prisons or police, because there was no crime. One of Dr. Bernard Jensen's highlights of that trip was staying as a guest of the Mir of Hunza's palace for 10 days.

Dr. Bernard Jensen visited the Caucasus Mountains in the USSR to meet a 153-year-old man who had stopped riding horseback a few years earlier only because of his doctor's orders. Dr. Bernard Jensen traveled to Vilacamba, Ecuador, where heart patients were able to recuperate so marvelously. Everywhere Dr. Bernard Jensen went, he brought back some new remedy or approach to integrate into the system he taught his patients.

Dr. Bernard Jensen received his Ph.D. at the age of 75 from the University of Humanistic Studies, San Diego, California.

Dr. Bernard Jensen retired from active chiropractic practice in 1978, and devoted himself to teaching, writing, and lecturing on the subjects of nutrition, rejuvenation, and iridology. Around this time, Dr. Bernard Jensen completed work on a two-hour feature film, titled *"World Search for Health,*

Happiness and Long Life," narrated by actor Dennis Weaver.

The Academy of Science in Paris awarded Dr. Bernard Jensen a medal in 1971 for exceptional services rendered to humanity. Also, in the same year, 1971, Dr. Bernard Jensen received an honorary doctorate from the Center for the Study of Human Sciences in Lisbon, Portugal.

At a ceremony in San Remo, Italy in 1973, Dr. Bernard Jensen was presented the Ignatz Von Peczely International Iridology Gold Medal by the World Congress of Scientific Medicine, an organization embracing many medical and health disciplines.

A congress of health professionals at Aixen Provence, France, in 1974, recognized Dr. Bernard Jensen with an award for his "valuable contribution in the field of iridology."

Then in 1975, the International Naturopathic Association honored Dr. Bernard Jensen for his service to mankind through his work in the fields of health, Iridology, and nutrition.

Knighted into the Order of St. John of Malta in 1978 for his humanitarian work in the field of health, Dr. Bernard Jensen was awarded the cross of St. John at a special ceremony in New York City. This Order is the oldest chivalric organization in the world, tracing its origin back to the time preceding the first Crusade.

In 1981, at the Fifth Annual Herb Symposium, the Agnes Arber Distinguished Service award was presented to Dr. Bernard Jensen for his contributions to the current "herb renaissance."

In 1982, the National Health Federation honored Dr. Bernard Jensen with its Pioneer Doctor of the Year award at its annual convention in Long Beach, California.

In 1982, Dr. Bernard Jensen traveled to Brussels, Belgium to accept the 1982 Dag Hammarskjold award of the Pax Mundi Academy, an international organization which presents annual awards to those in the arts and sciences who have made outstanding contributions in their fields. The award, in the category of scientific merit, was for "the exceptional services rendered to collective humanity... toward international cooperation and solidarity..." Dr. Bernard Jensen was personally congratulated on his award by U. S. Ambassador, Charles Price.

In 1988 Dr. Bernard Jensen held his 80th Birthday Celebration at the Town and Country Hotel in San Diego, California, where people came from all over the world to celebrate his 80 years of life and work in the holistic health field.

In 1993 he was presented with a PhD. in natural healing arts and sciences from Westbrook University, where his iridology course was part of the school curriculum.

In 1998 and 1999 Dr. Bernard Jensen received awards from the IIPA for his work in iridology.

In 2000 Dr. Bernard Jensen was awarded by Nature Sunshine an honorary award for his outstanding contributions to iridology and herbology before five thousand people.

On February 22, 2001 a month before his 93rd birthday, Dr. Bernard Jensen passed away at 92 years old.

The short biography above about Dr. Bernard Jensen is a small part of a larger biography I am writing about my grandfather's life. If you are interested in learning more I will be blogging and have more information at www.bernardjensen.org.

In the 21 lecture reprint booklets you'll see products or foods that might not be commonly found today. I left some things in to give the flavor of that time period and what he was thinking at that time. I also left in quotes or sayings from that era. I edited misspellings and grammatical errors. Overall, I feel that these booklets give down to earth advice and can still be regarded as basic knowledge in the mainstream health field today. A lot of his products are no longer available, but you can find what remains on my website, www.jensenholistichealth.com.

I hope you enjoy these lecture reprint booklets as much as I do and take them for what they are. If nothing else, a novelty and glimpse of the past. A simple approach from one of the early promoters of healthy living. Alongside such greats of that era like Paul Bragg, Jack LaLanne, Dr. Max Gerson, V.E. Irons, and Dr. Bronner at the beginning of a health revolution.

Jon D. Jensen

HOW TO REVITALIZE THE GLANDS

"My purpose is to serve and I must serve my purpose."

Bernard Jensen, Ph.D., D.C., N.D.

HOW TO BUILD A BETTER BODY
FROM YOUR KITCHEN

It is my sincere belief that we cannot be well and live a normal happy life unless we work to attain this happiness through three mediums: mental, spiritual, and physical. I do not think that a person, even though he may have a healthy body, can be really happy and live a successful life if he is sick in mind from worry.

These worries can stem from unhappiness in the home, an unhappy marriage, the wrong job, financial trouble, illness, or any other of the numerous sources of worry that plague people in this modern world. We must strive to overcome all of these worries and arrive at the place where we have, not only our health, but peace of mind and the happiness that comes from these two.

LEARN THE "RIGHT" PRINCIPLES

A person who knows nothing about spiritual principles is on the way when he starts seeking the right thing physically, because it is the desire, the incentive, the feeling for perfection in the physical that stimulates the same feeling and desire in the mental and spiritual work. You cannot separate these things.

We start our work with the physical, and the first step is the consideration of the food that we take into our body. Even though the food that we eat is for the physical body, it carries through to the brain and mind and to the soul as well.

We have three problems facing us today in getting good food for our family. First, there is the fact that the soil has become so depleted that we do not get the proper chemical and mineral elements in the food that we buy; secondly, the food that we get from the market is so refined and devitalized; and thirdly, the cooking procedures used in most of the homes really finish off the balance of chemical or mineral elements that may have been left in the food after the first two processes have robbed us.

The first two practices are rather difficult and will take a long range program to overcome, but the third problem we can certainly do something about, and right now!

RESPONSIBILITIES OF KITCHEN WORK

When we speak of kitchen preparation, we do not mean cooking entirely, even though there are a lot of people who think the kitchen is just for cooking foods. This is not entirely so. We should find ways of using kitchen implements to prepare foods so that when they are served to the family they have as much of the mineral and chemical elements left in them as possible.

We are responsible for the health of the family and this responsibility starts in the kitchen. The cook for the family is actually handling the future generation; the food we eat is going to walk and talk tomorrow. Surely, it is a responsibility that we cannot neglect. A wife may be responsible for cooking for her husband right onto an operating table, or even to the undertaker. Here is something to think about! She may also be responsible for the stiff joints of her family.

This is not only possible, but it is being done every day. Six million cases of arthritis and rheumatism in the United States last year started in the kitchen. Six million means nothing for we have touched on only arthritis and rheumatism. This six million does not include the four million cases of heart disease, the six hundred thousand that died from cancer, the seven hundred thousand that died of tuberculosis.

Every disease can get a good start in the kitchen. We can also stop disease right in the kitchen. What a responsibility for the mother, the cook, the food fancier or gourmet! The cook has your destiny in the palm of her hand. Talk about the Gods of Destiny!

FOOD EDUCATION IS NEEDED

Certainly, when we have been given such a beautifully and wonderfully created body, there is a way to maintain it. We recognize that three-fourths of the ailments in the hospital, and being treated by doctors, are caused by malnutrition because of the food that people are eating. We must educate people as to what the food they eat is going to do in the body. This is a serious matter. Experiments with diseased hogs prove that the diseases were cured when the hogs were fed a properly balanced diet. We have seen thoroughbred horses unable to walk because of improper food grown on improper soil. Thoroughbred or not, if the minerals and chemicals are not there, properly balanced, you will not walk and talk, you will not be a perfect human being. Beautiful racehorses are raised in Florida and California, but Kentucky is the most famous for its thoroughbred horses because of the Blue Grass, a product of an extremely rich soil.

In Switzerland people develop huge goiters because the rain washes the iodine into the sea, and the food grown there does not have enough iodine. In the United States there is a goiter belt where people develop goiters from eating food grown on that particular soil in their vicinity which is lacking in iodine.

I have worked experiments and know that by planting certain chemicals at the roots of certain plants we get double the development of the plant, double the strength and double the green running through the plant.

In one experiment we planted two rows of cabbages, one with all the chemicals at the roots, and as they grew they were green and beautiful, without a single worm, and yet only four feet away we planted a row of cabbages which did not have the chemical elements, and they were eaten up by disease and bugs.

If we are going to develop resistance in our bodies, we must start with the soil and the plant. Professor Albrecht of the University of Missouri Agricultural Department proves that he can grow better soybeans on soil which has the proper mineral elements.

WE NEED SOIL DOCTORS

Calcium in the leaves of the cabbage is almost double when the soil is rich in the chemical elements. In New York City, out of 5,000 cases tested, only two people were found to have enough calcium in their bodies. Again we come back to the soil problem. This is our big problem of the future! We need soil doctors, I know that when tomatoes have been grown in proper soil they can be sent to New York from California and returned to the original shipper, a total distance of 6,000 miles, and come back in perfect condition. They were sent ripe, and they stayed on a desk for one month and yet did not rot or spoil. That is what can be done when the soil is properly balanced and the plant grown in this type of soil.

THE PROCESSING OF FOOD

We now see that our first step in the right direction is in proper preparation of the soil in which we grow our food. The next step has to do with the processing of food.

When I say there is no Vitamin B in rice that has been polished, this is not just idle talk, yet rice is the best source of Vitamin B. Where is the Vitamin B in polished rice? It is in vitamin tablets that people are buying separately. How foolish this is when all you have to do is eat the natural brown rice. Stop and think. We eat the inside of grains, the acid part of the grains, and the part that has not even enough food for a weevil to live on. Mice and rats will not touch white flour or the inside of the grain.

Throughout history there were tribes that fed prisoners the inside of grains so they would be easy to overcome when they had to fight them. During this last war there was a law passed in England stating that no more white flour could be served their people. They were going to build better men and women.

When necessity comes we force ourselves into the right thing. We have the opportunity to do the right thing at all times, but we do not seem to see that the perfect thing should be done at all times and not just at the time of necessity.

SOME VITAL FOOD FACTS

We know that by feeding polished rice to pigeons, in four days they are so weak they die. Pigeons live two years on natural rice without any trouble whatever. The only difference between the four-day period of life and the two-year period of life is the outside hull of the rice.

Life does not mean much to some people except their own, but when others are depending on you, you owe them everything you can give them. This knowledge is not mine; I have not worked this out in my own head. This is for all of you. This is the experience of doctors. We have taken the inside of grains and made chicken feed out of it, and the chickens develop "droop wing". They cannot hold their wings in place. Many human beings are going around with the same condition.

STAFF OF LIFE — OR DEATH

The processing of flour is only one of the jobs that deprive us of the natural elements we need. We then use this devitalized flour to make bread or Danish pastry or many other things that suit our fancy. We salt, pepper, flavor, and when we stop we have made the food worse than ever. Bread could be the "staff of life," but the bread we get today in this country is the "staff of death." In my own practice, I have taken bread away from some people entirely, and this has done better than anything else I have done for them. When I cut bread from a patient's diet, no matter what their complaint may be, it helps them to better health.

In processing of foods, let us consider all products, not just the flour industry but other products, sweets, for instance. In them the vital or Life-Force elements are all, or nearly all, removed in the processing. Jello is 85% white sugar, and white sugar is devoid of practically everything, nutritionally speaking. It is the greatest calcium leech you can put in the body. It is definitely responsible for producing acids in the body which is the beginning of every disease, and it is definitely the cause of arthritis and rheumatism. So, if you eat it, what can you expect to have tomorrow or next year?

Just take one food, Jello. The only thing in it that is right is the gelatin. It is artificially flavored, artificially colored and surely the sugar that it has is not the real thing, so what have you that is real?

THE REAL AND THE UNREAL

There is very little that is real. Start with the sugar: we know there is less than 50% nourishment in white sugar, while there is some 98% nourishment in raw sugar. There are only two chemical elements that can be used for our good in white sugar, while there are fourteen that can be used for our good in raw sugar. Vitamin and mineral material can both be increased by using raw sugar or honey in a gelatin dessert. When we come to the artificial coloring and artificial flavoring, these are made from coal tar which acts as an irritant in the body. The package itself tells you that it contains less than 8% gelatin. It is far better to know what is real. Use less of the things which are bad for you. If you use real gelatin, using the real fruit juice and very little of even the natural sweeteners, you can make a dessert that is good for the body.

WE NEED KNOWLEDGE

If we knew the real thing to use, the most Godly thing, the thing we should have, we would certainly improve our health. All we need is knowledge.

The majority of appetizers and snacks are made of bad material to begin with, such as bacon rind, which has been burned to a crisp. We hear the radio blasting about it, so we accept it as something good. When we are able to recognize the real thing, we will have a knowledge of what is best for us. We should talk only of positive things, but so many negative things are thrown at us through advertising that it is difficult to combat. We should recognize that Cream of Wheat is bad, white sugar is bad, that there is not a single product of the Heinz 57 Varieties of stomachache that is good. Everyone has its toll; you pay in health.

Most people do not know that pepper is seventeen times more irritating to the liver than alcohol and that vinegar destroys red blood cells. If people knew these things they would not go right on using them and then go to a doctor to save themselves.

A still greater crime is for a doctor to treat your ailment and allow you to continue living the same way that caused your disease, without telling you, educating you in how to correct the trouble and how to avoid it in the future. Once this knowledge is universally known, it is going to be a crime to be sick, a crime to build the kind of diseases we are building today. You cannot say to a patient, "You got into this mess; you get out of it." The only way he can overcome his problem is by right living, by knowing how.

COFFEE AND CIGARETTES

Coffee and cigarettes are the two things doctors usually pick on as being bad for a person, but when I think of all the things we do during the day, there is very little that we do right. If we did 98% of the right things during the day, the 2% would be offset. The reason you cannot offset the bad effects of the caffeine is because you do not have the proper resistance. Rectal conditions have been improved in 15% of the cases in my practice by taking away coffee. Coffee is a powerful stimulant. I have seen people whose hearts have stopped, and by giving them an enema of coffee they have been brought back to life. If you are going to live on a heart stimulant, you will not live as long as you would by living a natural life. Any stimulant will kill you.

We know that every cigarette a person smokes takes two minutes off his life, and I am positive that if there were a way to tell what coffee does to a person, it would have the same drastic effect. In our ads and over the radio and on television they tell us they are adding Vitamin B to coffee. What mentality is going to use it? I do not blame the people who put it out; the people who use it are the ones at fault. The reason I say that is this: I know a gentleman in a flour concern who was responsible for spending $500,000.00 to educate people, telling them the value of whole wheat flour. After spending the amount, he found the sales still remained as they were with white flour 90% and whole wheat flour selling only 10%. When you talk to this man about humanitarian movements now he is not interested.

KITCHEN KNOWLEDGE

It would be wonderful for the housewife to have the knowledge so that she would know the best meal to serve her husband when he came home tired from work. She would know that if he is using his muscles a potassium broth would alkalinize the acid quicker than anything else. She would know that if he uses his mind, brain, and nervous system the mental foods, high in manganese, would alkalinize those tissues. If he had a stomach disturbance, digestive disturbance or lymphatic congestion a nice sodium broth would be used to alkalinize these conditions. How important this knowledge can be! I believe that with the knowledge I have I could train the average housewife in two weeks' time, and with this knowledge she could do more to eliminate disease than all the doctors, hospitals, and clinics we have in this country.

THE VALUE OF NATURAL FOODS

You may destroy the teeth of your children right in the kitchen. When I see a child of eleven with all of his teeth out and wearing false plates it makes one realize we must take the responsibility for our children's health. This is definitely so until the children reach an age when they can take care of themselves. We sometimes wonder just what we owe our family, but I do believe that in order to make the next generation better, we owe it to the children to see that they have the best start possible, and to get this we must start with natural foods. When we are using denatured and devitalized foods we know that a child cannot have the proper teeth, that rickets can develop, kidney and heart trouble can develop, also poliomyelitis, arthritis, and rheumatism. When you see reports from different schools that tell of curvatures of the spine, flat feet, eye trouble and ear trouble, and you realize that all of this comes from malnutrition, certainly it is the mother's job and mother's responsibility to see that the proper food is served.

I have handled cases where people with money have hired cooks to take care of the food. One of the first things I tell them is to either teach the cook to serve properly prepared meals or lay her off, otherwise I will not take the case. If they do not get the proper food into the stomach they cannot get well.

WHAT FOOD CAN DO FOR THE HEART

I can remember a case I had, a man with a very bad heart condition. This man's wife had heard my lectures and was very interested in getting some help for her husband. He had been under the care of doctors for the past six months, and he had been a bed case. In going over his case with him, I remember his telling me that there was only one job for me to do and that was, "Get me out of this bed." I said, "Well, there is only one thing you have to do, and that is to follow my advice. The first thing you will have to do is to eat as I tell you to." After we had worked out his diet program he told me no one in the house ate like that so who would prepare the food? The wife spoke up and said, "I'll see that it is done."

The first thing they did was lay off the cook who had been traveling with them for years. In six weeks' time this man was out of bed, was able to swim in the ocean, and to play nine holes of golf. He had been told that he would never be able to move into his new home which he was building in Texas. One day I received a call from him inviting me to a farewell dinner, as he was leaving to take up residence in that new home. As we sat down to the table I was impressed by the beautiful centerpiece which was a display of fresh fruits and vegetables. He told me, "In the past, when our food was cooked it was always without color and always heavily spiced, salted and peppered, but now that we are eating these natural foods our health has improved."

VITAMINS AND MINERALS ARE THE BASIS OF HEALING

Let us look at the basis of the healing business, vitamins and minerals. These are the basis, the block builders, our building stones; they are nerve and cell joiners and they have magnetic power. Vitamins and minerals have healing ability; they build quality as they go into every organ of our body and help rid us of disease. We certainly should bless food that goes into our bodies, but how much more of a blessing we would receive from natural food rather than from white bread, ghost bread, mashed potatoes, fried foods, doughnuts and coffee, pickles, and ice cream. Natural God-given food is a blessing in itself.

The man who must think and create will have a difficult time accomplishing this on a bowl of Cream of Wheat. You cannot expect a man to walk, to have the ability to accomplish, to push, to lift, if he is going to eat crullers and dumplings. It is impossible. WE know that we must have minerals. After all, if the foods have been deteriorated in processing and kitchen preparation, what can we hope to get out of it? If we expect good health, we are doomed to disappointment.

The body is made up of an ash weighing about five or six pounds. This is the mineral content of the body. It has been said we are only worth about ninety-eight cents, but we can buy out the drugstore, purchasing chemicals and minerals, but it takes more than just this to make a man.

VITAMINS ARE ESSENTIAL TO OUR HEALTH

Vitamins are an essential part of our health program and are not found in any worthwhile quantity in preserved, pickled, salted, peppered, processed, denatured, polished, and other over-processed or over-cooked foods. The average cook does not know that by putting soda in vegetables to keep them green she is starting stomach trouble in the one who eats those vegetables. She probably does not realize that she has to serve three times as much food to the same amount of nourishment from fried foods as she would if she served baked or roasted food. Truly, what the prophet has said, "We shall eat but we shall not be filled" is true.

The informed cook knows how to preserve foods with low heat, with very little sugar, using date sugar or honey. She knows ways of cold packing; she will preserve foods through freezing and will always do things the most natural way possible. She will bake, broil, and roast instead of frying and boiling and stewing her foods to death.

THE COOK CAN PRODUCE BEAUTY

The cook has the privilege of producing beauty, of improving the complexion, of putting weight on the body. What a privilege to know that she can be a sculptor right in the kitchen. It has been said that when you eat a doughnut, it is a minute in your mouth, four hours in your stomach and the rest of your life on your hips! Right in the kitchen we have the privilege of building the blood and resistance to disease. We know also that from the kitchen we can prevent doctor bills, that we can maintain perfect teeth in the family; we can start a child on the right diet; we can do away with fatigue, eliminate gas disturbances, and see to it that the family is not one of those contributing to the nine million dollars that is spent for laxatives each year. Knowledge is invaluable when we realize that in cases of skin disorders there are skin producing elements to take care of them, and that if the kidneys are not working properly there are foods that will stimulate kidney activity.

KIDNEY ACTIVATOR

Speaking of a kidney activator, one of the best is the use of watermelon juice, when used in the case of kidney stones. We have used it many times and find that we are able to dissolve and break down kidney stones through the use of this juice. The patient speaks of passing off a substance like sand through the urine when using watermelon juice. Use the red inside of the melon and the white rind and put it through a juicer or liquefier and strain it. Give the patient an eight ounce glass every two to three hours. For best results use this juice for two or three days. It is better to keep the patient in bed so that there is no irritation in the body or irritation to the stone, as it may be lodged in the ureter itself. Watermelon is very high in silicon, which is used to help eliminate infection in any part of the body. Silicon is one of the finest things we can use to cure boils on the body. An infection may set up when kidney stones irritate the kidney or the tubes they pass through, but if silicon is already there from the watermelon juice administered, it will help alleviate any infection that may set in. In this way we are using food as a medicine.

DON'T WASTE VITAMINS

For cooking, kitchen experts of the United State Department of Agriculture have established the following common sense rules:

1. Do not stir air into food while cooking.

2. Do not put food through a sieve while hot.

3. Do not use soda in cooking green vegetables.

4. In boiling foods, raise the temperature to the boiling point as rapidly as possible.

5. Use as little water as possible.

6. Do not use cooking processes such as stewing when shorter methods are feasible.

7. Do not throw away the water in which vegetables have been cooked. Use it in making gravies, sauces, and soups. (This is one of the most important of these rules.)

8. Do not fry foods valuable for their content of vitamins A, B, or C.

9. Prepare chopped fruit and vegetable salads just before serving.

10. Start cooking frozen foods while they are still frozen.

11. Serve raw frozen food immediately after thawing.

WE MUST SEEK THE RIGHT VALUES

Most of us reach a time in life when we must seek values. We try various things constantly to find out whether we can use them or not. It is wise to evaluate the equipment in your kitchen. We have not put the value on our kitchen that we should. We do not realize that this one room is the storehouse of health; that our future is there and that we are either going to raise a doctor bill from what comes out of that kitchen, or we are going to be in good health. Our values in life are distorted if we are going to measure this on the dollar basis. Health is one of our greatest achievements, and if we fail in this one thing, are we not falling short of one of the greatest values in life?

HAVE YOU TRIED THE RIGHT KIND OF EQUIPMENT?

The ordinary family will find that they have spent approximately $150 to $250 on their kitchen equipment. If I told you to throw out all this old-fashioned equipment, most of which cooks up only ill health for the family and go out and spent $250 for real health-giving kitchen equipment, you would probably think I was losing my mind. Yet, this is exactly what you should do for your family's health.

If you were told by some heart specialists that it would be necessary for you to purchase a machine costing $300 to overcome your heart condition, you probably could not get to the store fast enough to buy the machine.

When I tell you that by equipping your kitchen with a complete set of stainless steel cooking utensils, which would cost you less than the $300 and which would prevent you and other members of the family from developing the illness that would require large doctor bills, suffering, hospital bills, and the machine I spoke of, you are horrified.

Where is your sense of value? You may find that money has the least value of all the things you want, because money will not buy the things that will give you the greatest happiness in life. Ask any man who is blind. If he were rich he would trade every cent he had for his eyes.

MONEY CANNOT BUY HEALTH

There is no one who does not consider health the most valuable possession that he has. Money cannot buy health, and it cannot buy happiness. Knowledge is the only thing that can do that. Your knowledge is your greatest possession. Be the wise man; use the knowledge that is already here. You have had an introduction to it; strike out and use this knowledge with wisdom, put the proper value on it, and go to work.

It is important to realize that there is no lunch complete with just starches or just sandwiches, as you should not eat bread without having vegetables with it. Starches alone, when run through the intestinal tract, through these warm chambers, will become dehydrated and hard and constipating. The body cannot properly handle starches without having vegetable fibers with them. Vegetable fibers hold some of the liquid from the vegetables, and thus we avoid constipation. I do not approve of eating sandwiches consistently. A cold baked potato can be used in a lunch, and if seasoned with the right dressing it would take the place of bread. Use a small cup of rice pudding, a little barley or barley pudding combined with dried fruit.

Some people have an idea that these starches have to be eaten hot, but they can be eaten cold as well. In adding vegetables to lunches, use carrot stocks, celery sticks, sliced peppers. Peppers are even higher in Vitamin C than orange juice and grapefruit juice. So you see, we can get our vitamins in vegetables as well as in fruit. We can also add stuffed dates to a lunch, even stuffed prunes that have been soaked overnight. Stuff the prunes with nut butter or cheese, and you may add any of the other fruits that have been dried and that have been soaked up.

PARENTS SHOULD KNOW ABOUT RIGHT FOODS

All of us would bless our parents if we knew that they had given us a good body and kept it in good health until we were on our own. I know that most adults would have all their teeth today if their mothers had known what I know today and had used that knowledge.

Through a study of food we recognize that we can build a more perfect body. Foods that are old and coarse do not have the same vitality as young, fresh, and tender foods. Milk from a young goat has a higher sodium content and vitality which far surpasses the milk taken from an older goat. Calves cannot live on pasteurized milk; cats that live on pasteurized milk have bones that break, bad breath, and digestive disturbances. These are all interesting facts to know, and we can profit from this knowledge.

THE EFFECTS OF CONDENSED MILK

At Randleigh Farm in New York every animal fed on pasteurized milk died of a disease while the animals fed on raw milk were healthy. There have been volumes written, with pictures, graphs, and charts, showing that bone and muscle structure is far better, in animals fed on raw milk than in those living on pasteurized milk. The animals having the poorest hair, the poorest skin, and develop the smallest, scrawniest bodies, the poorest teeth, the most brittle bones are those fed on condensed milk.

The cooking process of boiling may take all the iodine from your foods. Remember the smell of cabbage when it is cooking? Do you know what that smell is? Actually it is vitamins and minerals escaping into the air—vitamins and minerals which are necessary to your body. Low heat cooking is necessary to keep the flavor and to keep these foods as near the natural thing as possible.

The man who discovered the cure for pellagra, which is a disease occurring when calcium and vitamins are lacking in the body, has been given the greatest nutritional prize in the country. The cure for pellagra is turnip greens. There is wonderful power, tone, and energy that comes from the proper amount of calcium in the body.

THE VALUE OF GREENS IN THE DIET

There is a group of people in Indo-China who die at the age of 125 with every tooth in their head. They have an ample supply of calcium in their body. They never have a child who has rickets. A child was born to a woman at the age of 85 years. One man was the head of the polo team at the age of 75 years. In the study of the diet of these people, we learned a secret you should never forget—60% of their diet is greens, the tops of vegetables. Greens live in sunshine, the very thing that controls the calcium in our bodies, and they will do more for the health of your family than any-thing else I can tell you. The green in the plant is the blood of the plant, and when it enters the human system it enters into the blood stream almost without pre-digestion.

In an experiment it was found that by taking all the blood from a rat and injecting the green from a living plant into the veins of the rat, it went right on living. That is how green compares with the blood in our bodies. You can forget other things but remember greens in your diet.

A GOOD DIET PROGRAM

A good diet program must include one starch a day, and that means starches that have good coating on them, those that are hard, that have resistance like hard Montana wheat, unpolished rice, wild oats and rice, steel cut oats, unpeeled barley, for these are the starches that have resistance and power to keep away disease within themselves and will help you build a body that is able to resist all disease.

You should have one good protein a day. If you are going to use meat, remember you must have lean meat and meat from a young animal. Use only white fish that has fins and scales; milk should be raw, from young animals, preferably warm. Try to get eggs that are from young chickens that have been eating lots of greens—the more greens the darker the yolk will be, and that is where the real vitamins and minerals are found.

VEGETABLES ARE A MUST

Include at least four vegetables and at least two fruits a day and remember in your combinations that if you have meat or proteins, have a little citrus fruit, tomato juice, grapefruit juice, or lemonade. When you have sweet fruits, starches are not allowed. It is better not to mix starches and proteins in one meal.

Start the day with fruit and milk. Have a starch at noon and protein at the evening meal with vegetables. Between meals use fruit, fruit juices, vegetable juices, tonics, and teas.

NUTS IN THE DIET

Grind nuts and make nut butters of them and you will find you will get more good out of them. The almond is the king of all nuts, and if we are going to get all of the protein out of it we must consider the easiest way to digest it. Blanch almonds and soak in pineapple juice, apple juice, or honey water. When soaked over a period of six to eight hours they will become soft, and your body will be able to absorb all the good from them almost immediately.

When nuts are not soaked they pass through the intestinal tract before we have a chance to absorb the nourishment that is in them. Most vegetarians are protein starved for this reason. They do not have the nuts prepared properly so that the body can digest them, and a weak system cannot get all of the protein out of nuts unless they have been soaked, made into nut butter, or flaked.

A VARIETY OF JUICES IS ESSENTIAL

Grape juice is slightly laxative, and very few people should use it continually, only on special occasions. Think of fig juice, prune juice, apple and pineapple juice. When we speak of juice we mean a variety of juices. When feeding oranges to a child, peel them and have him eat the pulp, as it is the easiest on the intestines and acts like a broom in cleaning out catarrh in the intestinal tract.

Try different kinds of vegetables. Parsley is one of the finest green vegetables. Parsley juice has ten times as much iron as lettuce. It is used for the kidneys and is good when used as an enema. Parsley juice can also be placed in the bath to get chlorophyll in the system.

CHLOROPHYLL IN THE BATH

Few people assimilate all of the food taken into the intestinal tract. If people really knew how much we absorb through the skin they would recognize that even a chlorophyll bath should be indulged in occasionally. By using parsley juice or chlorophyll directly in the bath we have shown definite results of improving the blood count. You may also use parsley juice or chlorophyll directly on the skin. Doctors are using chlorophyll salves in cases of ulcers, leg ulcers, and are even using this green top chlorophyll material for rectal sores and rectal conditions. It is mixed with glycerin suppositories. This green is the finest healer we have. Many cases of eczema, pimples, breaking out of the skin can be helped by using this green juice directly on the skin.

Barley gruel is soothing to the stomach and should be used when a person is tired and not capable of digesting a heavy meal. Soothing broths and soups always set well on the stomach in a tired body.

THE VALUE OF TEAS

Mint tea has the property of driving out gas and relaxing the stomach; oats and oat straw tea carry the property of feeding silicon to the body for the care of veins in the legs, feet or hands, and it gets rid of dry skin. Bran tea is very high in silicon and will help people who want to get the gloss back into the hair and help a poor skin condition.

FISH FOR HIGH STRUNG PEOPLE

For the high strung, excitable person clam juice and fish broths are helpful to the nerves. In extreme cases cook the bones of fish as they are rich in phosphorous and other brain and nerve elements that are needed by the system. We cook the bones of the animal and also the head and fins of the fish as they, too, are especially good for the person who wants to build up the brain and the nervous system.

A GOOD BLOOD TONIC

Limes are wonderful to neutralize the condiments found in some prepared foods. Lime juice and whey make a good tonic for the blood of a person who has a quick temper. Whey is also one of the best things to take care of any hardness in the body. It is a great dissolver and one of the highest sodium foods we can use. It is especially good to use in all digestive disturbances. We find that in arthritis, neuritis, pleurisy, lung catarrh, or any condition of the body where we want to neutralize any acid, whey is the best thing to use, whether it be from cow's milk or goat milk.

WHAT SODIUM DOES FOR YOU

Sodium is the chemical element that keeps joints limber, pliable, active, movable, and sodium is the element we call the youth element. We could go still further and use whey as an enema to add the extra lactic acid that the acidophilus bacterial needs in the intestinal tract.

The gizzard of an animal is very high in sodium. Make a gizzard broth of chicken gizzards and use as a dissolver in the body.

IODINE FOODS

The over-emotional person should use iodine foods such as sea plant foods and different fish that contain iodine. Turtle broth is one of the finest things to feed the glands and nerves to bring them back to normal. Black cherry juice is high in iron. Mix cherry juice with parsley juice, and you have the finest thing to overcome anemia that I can recommend. Muffins made with yellow corn meal give us a supply of magnesium which is necessary for bowel tone. When making muffins, add a little rice polishings.

There is no one so well but that he should add a few of the products found in the health food store to his diet.

A FEW IDEAS

Make your own ice cream with fresh eggs and gelatin. There are many combinations you can make using honey, bananas, nuts of different varieties, or raisins. So many good things can be made into ice cream and sherbets, and these can be health builders.

Make waffles, which are more desirable than hot cakes or pancakes, and serve with maple syrup instead of cheap syrups and white sugar products. You must be careful of combinations for it is in the flour and sugar combinations that we develop gases and intestinal disorders.

Fruit alone is not enough for the small child's breakfast. Select a good whole wheat cereal such as cracked wheat, Seven in One, or ground barley, which are all good. In preparing the cereal, start with cold water and just simmer until every particle is separated. Extreme heat in the cooking is the only reason every particle seems not to separate, holding together in a mass and becoming hard to digest. If possible, use distilled water, strained rainwater, or spring water in preference to city water. City water destroys the iodine in foods for the chlorine use in the purification of the water is an iodine destroyer. Iodine, which is water soluble, dissolves in steam.

POSTURE AFFECTS THE THYROID GLAND

The Thyroid gland is the most abused gland today because of bad posture. We sleep with a pillow and create pressure on the thyroid gland. Then we are emotionally upset; we fight; we nag; we become disturbed, and all of this disturbs the thyroid gland.

We also abuse the thyroid gland through cooking the iodine out of food. See to it that your family gets a proper amount of iodine. Onions should be used plentifully in the kitchen during the winter, for it is one of the best cold preventatives and aids in building up resistance to catarrhal producing germ life.

WHAT TO DO FOR FLU

In cases of flu or bad cold, one of the best things to use is a lemon that has been baked in the oven for a period of over twenty minutes. After it has been baked, cut the lemon in half and put into a glass of hot water and drink slowly, go to bed and cover yourself and perspire.

Clabbered milk is a good food to use to build up a normal intestinal flora. Clabber must be kept in a cool place until you are going to use it. Cover milk you wish to clabber with a closely woven cloth or double thickness of cheese cloth and contact with air will clabber it. Do not drink sour milk as it is not good for you, but when milk becomes clabbered it is good for you. It takes about two days for the acidophilus to develop. Clabber can only be made from raw milk; you cannot clabber pasteurized milk — it will turn green.

Any man who would spend his life getting rid of pasteurized milk would do much toward getting rid of disease in the United States today. Look at this country today. We are talking care of sick people at a cost of $1,500,000, and we do not have enough beds to take care of the insane people. There will not be enough sane people to take care of the insane people in another eighty years. This is a disgraceful condition.

Sickness should be a thing of the past! The time will come when people will have the proper knowledge and use it, and then it will be a disgrace to be sick.

RAW GOAT'S MILK

Raw goat's milk has one hundred times as much fluorine and builds harder enamel on the teeth than cow's milk. In fact, goat's milk contains more fluorine than any food you can take. Dentists recognize this and have recorded this fact in the Dentists' Journal. Schools of dentistry are the first to put a dietary program in their college courses. The University of California has added a course in nutrition. Slowly people are being educated on diet truths.

Once I was a foreman at a creamery, and at another time I had forty goats in a raw milk dairy. I refused to serve milk at my sanitarium when it had been pasteurized. I have five sons living on this raw milk. Parents are so frightened when the word "poliomyelitis" is mentioned. I wonder too, some-times, whether I should take the chance. I do not know exactly how many cases of poliomyelitis there are in the country, possibly 10,000. Then I wonder if I would rather have my child be one of the unfortunates—of the 6,000,000 wracked with pain from arthritis and rheumatism or one of the sufferers of heart disease—or one of the 10,000 unfortunate sufferers of undulant fever. I, personally, would rather take the chance of using raw milk than using pasteurized milk which leads to these other diseases.

IT'S YOUR DECISION

You have to decide whether you are going to build good resistance or poor resistance. Are you going to build your body on coffee and doughnuts and drink unfit milk, or are you going to build up a good body, strong enough to throw off diseases?

We are the most fearful race on the face of the earth. There is not a week that goes by without a "Prevent" something week. What about a "Good Health Week?" If you asked, "How do you prevent infantile paralysis, tuberculosis, and other diseases?" I would definitely say, "Stop using pasteurized milk." As it is my considered opinion that infantile paralysis is due to pasteurized milk. I sincerely believe this, for most cases show that patients lack fluorine, and fluorine is the one chemical element that goes up in steam when milk is pasteurized. All children are going to develop illnesses from a lack of fluorine if we continue giving them only pasteurized milk.

There have been many articles printed in recent years, such as, "Are We Starving to Death?," "Hidden Hunger," "Hidden Famine," and these make us wonder if we are actually committing suicide right in our own homes, in our kitchens by the way we prepare the food we eat.

SOME FACTS ON CANCER

The Literary Digest quotes that one out of every four women have cancer. In China 60% of the cancers are found in men's throats. When we find that the Chinese women do not have so much cancer of the throat, we wonder what causes this difference. We believe this difference can be found in the fact that in

China the men sit down to the table and eat first, so they eat their rice when it is very hot. By the time the women sit down the rice has cooled off, and we believe this fact could be a contributing factor to the prevalence of cancer of the throat among men in China. Build the body using food at body temperature; never use extremely hot or cold foods.

I am sure that everyone wants to do the right thing so that he and all the members of his family will enjoy abundant health. We can sum it all up by saying buy fresh foods, cook them over low heat in clean stainless steel cookware that seals in all of the vitamins and minerals while cooking, and serve at moderate temperature. Use the natural qualities found in natural foods as your medicines, as well as for your taste treats. You will find that you will not need a doctor and that you will enjoy yourself to the utmost, for you will have REAL HEALTH.

VEGETABLE JUICES

I think everyone should drink vegetable juices. Use at dinner time as a cocktail or between meals instead of water. Vegetable juices are truly a filtered water, and they are most electrical in their effect in the body. They are dissolvers, "light" water that keeps the body limber, active, elastic in its activities.

A SPECIAL ONE-DAY SUGGESTION

Everyone should fast one day a week or at least go on juices one day a week. They can be vegetable juices, fruit juices, or both. This gives the body a day of rest as far as the intestinal tract is concerned. Also rest physically and mentally. This helps the body to repair broken down tissues. It is during rest that we can best build a new body.

SPECIAL SUGGESTIONS FOR LIVER AND GALL BLADDER TROUBLES

Liver and gall bladder troubles are usually found to be at the base of most people's troubles, whether they suffer from colitis, high blood pressure, rheumatism, arthritis, catarrh, acidity, or what. One of the best suggestions for cleansing the gall bladder and liver is to drink dandelion tea or a more palatable drink made from beet greens. One cannot take a finer liver or gall bladder cleanser than beet greens. They may be taken as a juice, a broth, or as a cooked vegetable. They may be taken daily or every other day for a month.

FLETCHERIZING OUR FOODS

We have heard much about Fletcherizing our foods. They should be well chewed so as to break down all the fibers and get more of the vitamins and minerals that are so necessary to good health. Fletcherizing aids the mechanical work of digestion and prevents overeating. We must take time to chew our foods well, therefore, if we want to have good health.

There are certain basic necessities for every health kitchen in the way of utensils and staples to have on the shelf. I have found the following list very helpful to the person who really wants to live the health way.

WORKING UTENSILS

Stainless steel cooking utensils. Hand grinder that grates and shreds, called the ricer. Chopping bowl with chopping knives, Vegetable juicer, and Vegetable liquefier.

PROTEINS

Soybeans ground for butter or for making patties; Lentils, ground for making patties and for thickening soups. High grade burr ground whole wheat flour for all cooking and baking purposes and for thickening soups (wheat is not only a good source of natural starch but contains very high grade amino acids found in protein.) Sesame seeds. Almond nut butter (a good meat substitute). Raw peanut butter, rich in minerals, protein and carbohydrates. (Not good for reducing.)

STARCHES

Banana powder, Jackson's Meal, Bragg's Meal, Hauser's Meal, Deaf Smith County Cereal, Rye Crisp, Orowheat Bread, Yellow Cornmeal, brown rice, barley, raw peanut butter, soya flour, ground coconut, any whole wheat bread made with burr ground, high grade wheat. (Some grist mills make their own high grade breads and muffins, enriching them with wheat germ and skim milk solids.) Potato meal and powder, sesame seeds, flaxseed meal which is rich in vitamin F.

SUPPLEMENTS

(For enriching drinks, soups, etc.) Skim milk powder, Black strap molasses, Rice Polishings, Flaxseed Meal (for vitamin F), Wheat Germ, Yeast Flakes, Sunflower Seeds, Ground Sesame Seeds,

Powdered and coarsely ground Coconut, Vegetable Broth Powder.

TEAS

Mint Tea, Alfalfa Mint Tea, Flaxseed Tea, Oat Straw Tea, Shave Grass Tea, Strawberry Leaf Tea, Huckleberry Tea, Fenugreek Tea, Bran Tea.

COFFEE SUBSTITUTES

Hollywood Cup and Kevo.

SWEETENERS

Honey, Raw Sugar and Date Sugar.

DRIED SWEET FRUITS

Dates, raisins, figs (these are nice to give the family instead of pastry sweets.) Prunes are good as a sweet or a regulator. When no fresh fruits are to be had, properly stewed dried apples, apricots, or pears are good substitutes.

HERBS, SPICES, SEASONINGS

Garlic Powder, Celery Seeds, Bay Leaves, Rosemary, Basil, Dill, Dulce, Lemon Powder, Sage, Paprika, Caraway, Thyme, Fennel, Chervil, Parsley.

Your Health Food Store will be glad to help supply your kitchen with the best foods possible, they are health-minded and are in business to serve you. No one should buy in a grocery store until he knows how and what to buy. Be careful of preservatives, foods that have been colored, denatured, and unnaturally treated, etc.

Let me list what I consider the five best starches and the five best proteins. The five best starches are: baked potato, banana (well ripened or baked), barley, brown rice, yellow corn meal.

The five best proteins are: meat is considered the best protein (this includes fowl and fish); raw milk; eggs, cheese (any cheese that breaks), cottage cheese; almond nut butter or flaked almonds; legumes.

HOW TO GAIN WEIGHT

Use liquefied salads, always adding soybean powder, egg yolk, or a banana. Dried fruits added to any liquefied drink, and taken between meals, helps in gaining weight. Work for good health first, before thinking of gaining weight. It is better to be healthy and thin than "normal weight" and sick.

HOW TO LOSE WEIGHT

If you want to lose weight, you might consider going on a low calorie diet for a short time, which we will outline here. However, notice that the foods you eat must be natural. You are bound to lose weight if you faithfully carry out the following diet regime for one week.

FIRST DAY		
BREAKFAST	Calories	Total
Tomato juice (1 – glass)	50	
Berries in season (1 cup)	60	
Whole wheat toast (2 slices)	120	

Butter (1/2 pat)	40	
Black coffee, tea, or substitute	10	280

LUNCHEON	Calories	Total
Cottage cheese (4 oz.) w/ chopped chives or green onions	120	
Tossed salad: lettuce (4 leaves) cucumber (1/4), celery and tops (4 stalks), chopped parsley (1/4 cup), tomato, honey, and lemon dressing (1 tsp. ea.)	95	
Skim milk (1 glass)	85	
Grapes (med bunch)	90	390

DINNER	Calories	Total
Consommé (1 cup)	30	
Lean broiled steak (6 oz.)	200	
Steamed vegetables, 1 leafy (2 1/2 cup)	70	
Butter (1/2 pat)	40	
Skim milk (1 glass)	90	430
Calorie total for first day		1100

SECOND DAY

BREAKFAST	Calories	Total
Pineapple juice (1 glass unsweet)	140	
1 egg, poached or boiled	80	
Fresh fruit, or 1 small serving soaked dried fruit	100	
Skim milk (1/2 glass)	45	
Black coffee, tea, or substitute	10	375

LUNCHEON	Calories	Total
Vegetable plate: spinach or Swiss chard string beans, shredded beets crook neck squash cooked with onion (1 cup each), baked potato	195	
Butter (1 pat)	80	
Skim milk or buttermilk (1/2 gl.)	45	
Cherries (20)	70	390

DINNER	Calories	Total
Bouillon (1 cup)	30	
Broiled ground round steak (6 oz. mixed in wheat germ and garlic salt)	210	
Shredded salad of cabbage (1/2 cup), carrot (1 med) apply (1/2), served with	95	335

lemon and honey dressing (1/2 tsp. ea.)		
Calorie total for second day		1100

THIRD DAY		

BREAKFAST	Calories	Total
Prune or apple juice (1 glass)	140	
Fruit plate of sliced orange berries (1/2 cup) soaked dried figs (3) melon balls (1/2 cup) sprinkled with banana flakes (1 tbsp.)	230	
Black coffee, tea, or substitute	10	380

LUNCHEON	Calories	Total
Green pepper omelet (1 egg, ½) green pepper	90	
Salad of sliced tomato, romaine lettuce (1/4 head)	60	
Whole grain toast (1 slice)	60	
Butter (1/2 pat)	40	
Skim milk or buttermilk (2/3 gl.)	55	305

DINNER	Calories	Total

Vegetable broth (1 cup)	50	
Broiled halibut steak (4 oz.) served lemon and parsley	200	
Steamed green peas (1/3 cup) and brussels sprouts (5)	60	
Butter (1/2 pat)	40	
Salad of: Lettuce (4 leaves) celery (1 stalk), cucumber (1/4 med.), green onion (1) lemon and oil dressing (1 tsp. ea.)	65	415
Calorie total for third day		1100

FOURTH DAY

Use diet regime above for First Day.

FIFTH DAY

Use diet regime above for Second Day

SIXTH DAY

Use diet regime above for Third Day.

SEVENTH DAY

Use diet regime above for First Day.

ADULTERATED FOODS

Pickles, catsup, canned foods such as canned meats, canned fruits, canned vegetables; sauces or spiced foods, baker's bread, smoked pork, baked hams, bacon, corned beef and cabbage, manufactured ice cream, manufactured pies and cakes, syrups of all kinds.

DISEASE-PRODUCING FOODS

Fruit flavorings, fruit colorings, any food that has been burned, scorched, fried or boiled; jams, marmalades and jellies put up in white sugar, confectionery, white flour products, colored candies, soda pop, cola drinks, cocoa, beer, salted fish, pasteurized process cheese, pasteurized milk, all alcoholic drinks, soda biscuits, salt biscuits, any stimulant, tea, coffee, spiced sauces, pork, fried foods and pastries of all kinds, mineral waters, concentrated or very rich foods, rancid butter, patent medicines, synthetic vitamins, sugared drinks.

OTHER BOOKLETS BY DR. JENSEN

1. HOW TO ENJOY BETTER HEALTH FROM NATURAL REMEDIES

2. HOW TO RELAX AND RELIEVE TENSION

3. HOW TO REVITALIZE YOUR GLANDS

4. A NEW SLANT ON HEALTH AND BEAUTY—SLANT BOARD

5. A HEALTH PATTERN TO LIVE BY

6. HOW TO BUILD A BETTER BODY FROM YOUR KITCHEN

7. HOW THE BREATH OF LIVE SUSTAINS YOU

8. PHYSICAL, MENTAL AND SPIRITUAL BALANCE

9. DEVELOPING INWARD CALM

10. THE NEED FOR A NEW ATTITUDE

11. THE HEART AND THE CIRCULATORY SYSTEM

12. THREE STEPS TO THE HIGHER LIFE (Part I)

13. THREE STEPS TO THE HIGHER LIFE (Part II)

14. THREE STEPS TO THE HIGHER LIFE (Part III)

15. HEALTH FOR OUR CHILDREN

16. SPECIAL FOODS FOR SPECIAL NEEDS

17. LETS BEGIN AT THE BEGINNING

18. YOUR LOVE LIFE

19. INTESTINAL DISORDERS & FASTING & ELIMINATIVE DIETS

20. VOL. I — SECRETS I CAN SHARE WITH YOU

21. VOL. 11 — MORE SECRETS I CAN SHARE WITH YOU

MEET THE ORIGINAL AUTHOR

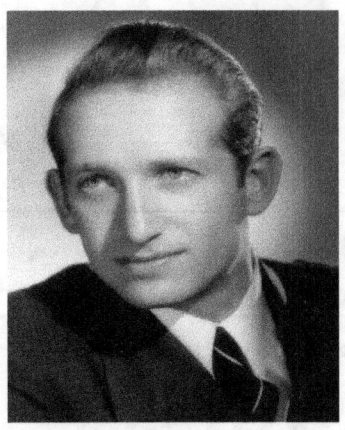

(From the back of the booklet)

Bernard Jensen, D.C, N.D., Nutritionist of Los Angeles, Calif. Born in Stockton, Calif, in 1908.

Possessing a convincing philosophy that would credit much older practitioners, Bernard Jensen, D.C, Lecturer and Teacher of Right Living, acquired from the beginning of his studies the vision "that Nature does all the healing." He believes doctors can only work with natural laws. His work is sane, up-to-date, practical, and teaches a balanced "how-to-live" regime.

At only 18, Dr. Jensen began studies with the West Coast Chiropractic College, Oakland, Calif. At 21 he began his practice of chiropractic in that city and has been practicing that science ever since. Widely traveled, he has been honored with post-graduate degrees from the National College in Chicago and the American School of Naturopathy, New York. He studied methods of the Battle Creek Sanitarium, of Tilden's School of Fasting in Denver. At an early age he was teaching his "How-to-live" methods to professional groups.

For 50 years. Dr. Jensen has led a most strenuous life, lecturing, radio broadcasting, and directing his own health center in Escondido, California.

His current plans include Radio and TV guest appearances, a nationwide tour, and more contributions to Iridology and color, with new works planned in both areas. Dr. Jensen's The Science and Practice of Iridology has brought him international acclaim and is currently being translated into Spanish. Nine more books are in various stages of production, including his spiritual masterpiece. Arise and Shine, and color book.

HIDDEN VALLEY HEALTH RANCH

Comfortable Accommodations

The accommodations are gaily decorated and furnished with every comfort—restful beds, spacious closets, and individually controlled heat. Each room will assure you a pleasant stay and a full night's sleep every night. Every attempt is made to make you as comfortable as possible. Accommodations are available at various rates to suit you.

Experience a new way of life, a non-demanding, relaxing, revitalizing way of living. Nestled in rolling country and continually blessed by pure fresh air, the ranch stretches over 200 acres of nature's artistry.

Your Hidden Valley vacation, or weekend, may well become a recurring part of your recreational plans. It is here that we make the best use of nature...organically grown food, exercise, pure water, and the right mental attitude all contribute to a vacation of unsurpassed value. Sun worshippers will enjoy the pool area or a leisurely walk around the ranch and hills can satisfy the desires of strollers, walkers, or hardy hikers.

About the Author

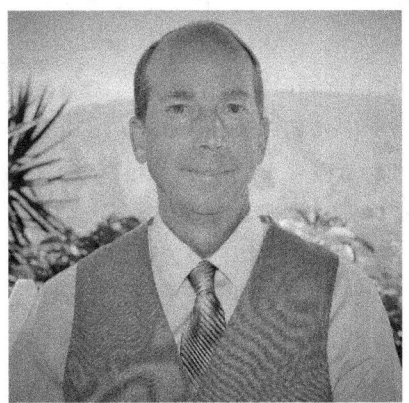

Jon Jensen, Iridologist, CMH, has been involved in holistic health for over 30 years with experience in Iridology, nutrition, and personal self-development. Jon started taking classes in Iridology and nutrition from his grandfather, the late Dr. Bernard Jensen, in 1980. Dr. Bernard Jensen is generally regarded throughout North America as the forefather of Iridology. Jon filled numerous roles over the years and participated in his grandfather's many classes and projects. Jon was involved in research for his grandfather's books, helping to pioneer a new way of iris analysis using the computer, and assisting with seminars.

Jon's mission is to educate people on the basic tenants of health and nutrition that his grandfather taught throughout his lifetime as a holistic health practitioner. Basics like the importance of a plant-based diet, regular exercise, proper sleep/rest, taking care of the bowel and more. Throughout his travels he searched for the longest living humans and wanted to know why they lived so long.

In 1995 Jon stayed by his grandfather's side after Dr. Bernard Jensen became paralyzed from the waist down from a car accident. Jon was right there every day of his grandfather's plan to walk again. With a big sign on the wall in front of Dr. Jensen's bed where he could see it every day that said, "LUCKY BOY". Every day consisted of many different healing modalities and supplements. Jon would travel to the Hidden Valley Health Ranch in the early morning and watch while Apolinar, Dr. Jensen's main ranch worker, milked the goat for Dr. Jensen's fresh morning goat milk drink. Jon would drive his grandfather and grandmother Marie to Los Angeles twice a week for chiropractic adjustments and frequency therapy, treating the whole body, mind, and spirit, and being involved in every aspect of what the doctors called a **"Miracle"—as his grandfather walked again on his own.** Jon is writing more on the entire recovery process and will publish it through Amazon.

After his grandfather's recovery, Jon shifted his attention to additional training by taking classes with some of the prominent leaders in the fields of Sclerology with Dr. Leonard Mehlmauer, Rayid (emotional iridology) with Denny Johnson, European based integrated iridology with Dr. Ellen Tart-Jensen as well as animal iridology with Dr. Mercedes Colburn. Jon attended Kalos© classes with Dr. Valerie Seeman-Gersch learning about Transformational Healing methods.

Jon was President of the Escondido Chapter of Chamber Toastmasters and enjoys speaking to groups.

Jon wrote an article for The Price-Pottenger Nutrition Foundation Journal on Animal Iridology and Nutrition. Jon has given presentations at: Holistic Health Fairs, Expo's, Herb Shops, Churches and Health Food Stores.

Jon is currently Executive Director at the "Live Pure Kids" foundation in Arizona. Jon works closely with Gavin Tucker the President/Founder, and Jackie Morales, Vice President.

The Live Pure Kids Foundation

Mission Statement: To change the world for our next generation starting from within.

Vision Statement: With the support of parents, families and the community, educating all kids through an organic plant-based mindfulness yoga lifestyle, we are giving our next generation the tools of today to be the world leaders of tomorrow.

www.livepurekids.com

Jon recently published a nutrition book called, *"A Simple Guide to Healthy Living"* along with the 21 Dr. Jensen Booklet series and they are available for purchase on Amazon.

For more information Jon can be found at www.jensenholistichealth.com
www.bernardjensen.org

www.ingramcontent.com/pod-product-compliance
Lightning Source LLC
Chambersburg PA
CBHW071247280526
45788CB00004B/1616